The Vibrant Dash Diet Cookbook

Lose weight and Stay Healthy with these 50 Delicios Dishes

Natalie Puckett

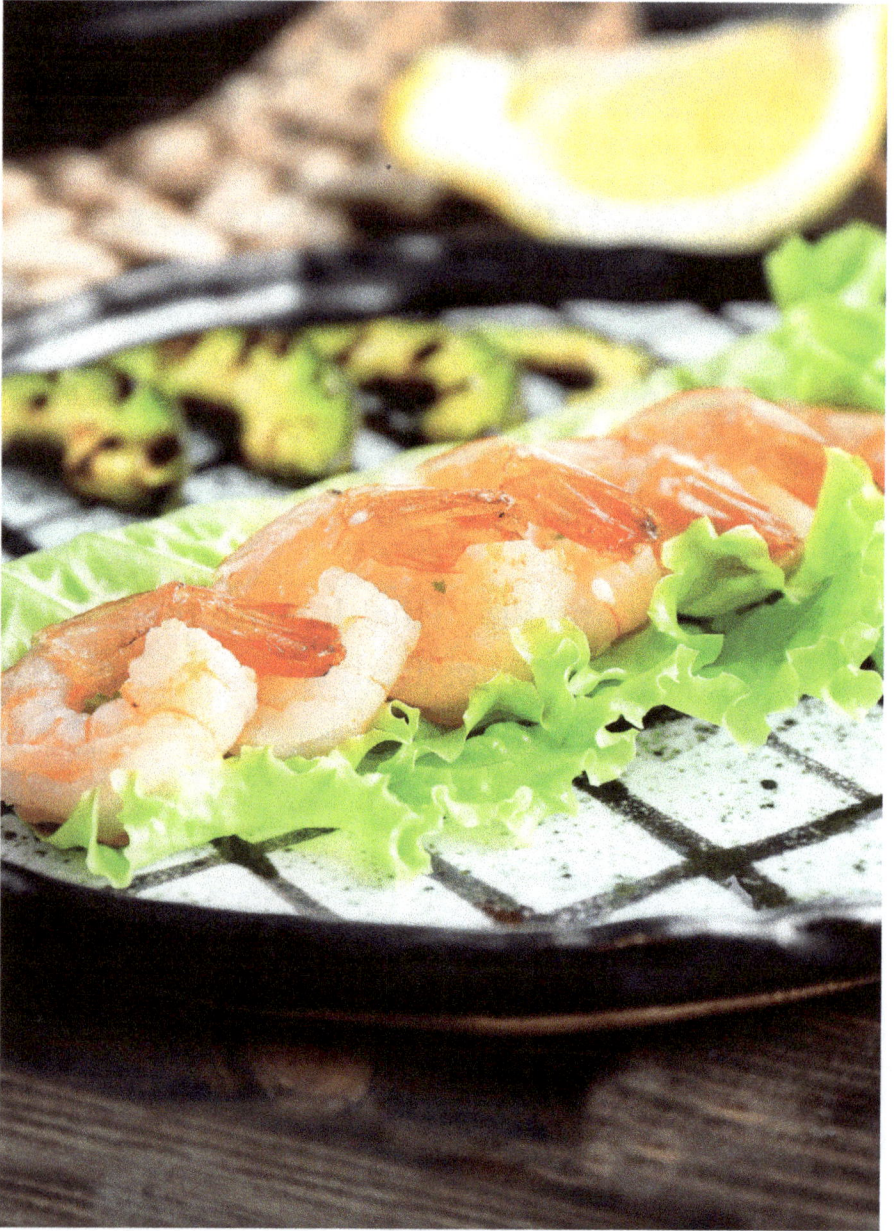

Table of Contents

SHRIMP AND AVOCADO PLATTER 5

CALAMARI 7

HEARTY DEEP-FRIED PRAWN AND RICE CROQUETTES.....................9

GROUND TURKEY MINI MEATLOAVES... 13

TURKEY AND BROWN RICE STUFFED PEPPERS 15

GRILLED TEQUILA CHICKEN WITH PEPPERS 17

ORANGE-ROSEMARY ROASTED CHICKEN 19

HONEY CRUSTED CHICKEN.. 21

ITALIAN CHICKEN AND VEGETABLE..24

CORN SPREAD..26

MOROCCAN LEEKS SNACK 28

THE BELL PEPPER FIESTA... 30

SPICED UP PUMPKIN SEEDS BOWLS...32

MOZZARELLA CAULIFLOWER BARS 34

TOMATO PESTO CRACKERS 36

GREEN DELIGHT..39

GUILT FREE LEMON AND ROSEMARY DRINK.............................. 41

STRAWBERRY AND RHUBARB SMOOTHIE 43

VANILLA HEMP DRINK 45

YOGURT AND KALE SMOOTHIE..47

BABY POTATOES...49

CAULIFLOWER CAKES 51

TENDER COCONUT AND CAULIFLOWER RICE WITH CHILI 53

APPLE SLICES 55

THE EXQUISITE SPAGHETTI SQUASH 57

VANILLA SWEET POTATO PORRIDGE 60

A NICE GERMAN OATMEAL..62

VERY NUTTY BANANA OATMEAL..64

COOL COCONUT FLATBREAD 67

PERFECT HOMEMADE PICKLED GINGER GARI 69

AVOCADO AND BLUEBERRY MEDLEY 71

HEALTHY ZUCCHINI STIR FRY 73

GREEK LEMON CHICKEN BOWL 75

CHILLED CHICKEN, ARTICHOKE AND ZUCCHINI PLATTER 77

CHICKEN AND CARROT STEW.. 79

TASTY SPINACH PIE 81

MESMERIZING CARROT AND PINEAPPLE MIX 84

ETHIOPIAN CABBAGE DELIGHT..86

THE VEGAN LOVERS REFRIED BEANS 88

COOL APPLE AND CARROT HARMONY..90

MAC AND CHOKES 92

BAY SCALLOP CHOWDER... 95

SALMON AND VEGETABLE SOUP.. 97

GARLIC TOMATO SOUP 99

MELON SOUP...101

SPRING SALAD 102

HEARTY ORANGE AND ONION SALAD.. 104

GROUND BEEF BELL PEPPERS 106

FOILED FISH... 108

BRAZILIAN SHRIMP STEW...110

Shrimp and Avocado Platter

Serving: 8

Prep Time: 10 minutes

Cook Time: nil

Ingredients:

2 green onions, chopped

2 avocados, pitted, peeled and cut into chunks

2 tablespoons cilantro, chopped

1 cup shrimp, cooked, peeled and deveined Pinch of pepper

How To:

1.   Take a bowl and add cooked shrimp, avocado, green onions, cilantro, pepper.

2.   Toss well and serve.

3.   Enjoy!

Nutrition (Per Serving)

Calories: 160

Fat: 2g

Net Carbohydrates: 5g

Protein: 6g

Calamari

Serving: 4

Prep Time: 10 minutes +1-hour marinating

Cook Time: 8 minutes

Ingredients:

2 tablespoons extra virgin olive oil

1 teaspoon chili powder

½ teaspoon ground cumin

Zest of 1 lime

Juice of 1 lime

Dash of sea sunflower seeds

½ pounds squid, cleaned and split open, with tentacles cut into ½ inch rounds

tablespoons cilantro, chopped

tablespoons red bell pepper, minced

How To:

1.   Take a medium bowl and stir in olive oil, chili powder, cumin, lime zest, sea sunflower seeds, lime juice and pepper.

2.   Add squid and let it marinade and stir to coat, coat and let it refrigerate for 1 hour

3.   Pre-heat your oven to broil.

4.   Arrange squid on a baking sheet, broil for 8 minutes turn once until tender.

5.   Garnish the broiled calamari with cilantro and red bell pepper.

6.   Serve and enjoy!

Nutrition (Per Serving)

Calories: 159

Fat: 13g

Carbohydrates: 12g

Protein: 3g

Hearty Deep-Fried Prawn and Rice Croquettes

Serving: 8

Prep Time: 25 minutes

Cook Time: 13 minutes

Ingredients:

2 tablespoons almond butter

½ onion, chopped

ounces shrimp, peeled and chopped

2 tablespoons all-purpose flour

tablespoon white wine

½ cup almond milk

tablespoons almond milk

cups cooked rice

1 tablespoon parmesan, grated

1 teaspoon fresh dill, chopped

1 teaspoon sunflower seeds

Ground pepper as needed

Vegetable oil for frying

tablespoons all-purpose flour

1 whole egg

½ cup breadcrumbs

How To:

1.   Take a large skillet and place it over medium heat, add almond butter and let it melt.

2.   Add onion, cook and stir for 5 minutes.

3.   Add shrimp and cook for 1-2 minutes.

4.   Stir in 2 tablespoons flour, white wine, pour in almond milk gradually and cook for 3-5 minutes until the sauce thickens.

5.   Remove white sauce from heat and stir in rice, mix evenly.

6.   Add parmesan, cheese, dill, sunflower seeds, pepper and let it cool for 15 minutes.

7.   Heat oil in large saucepan and bring it to 350 degrees F.

8.   Take a bowl and whisk in egg, spread breadcrumbs on a plate.

9.   Form rice mixture into 8 balls and roll 1 ball in flour, dip

in egg and coat with crumbs, repeat with all balls.

10.   Deep fry balls for 3 minutes.

11.   Enjoy!

Nutrition (Per Serving)

Calories: 182

Fat: 7g

Carbohydrates: 21g

Protein: 7g

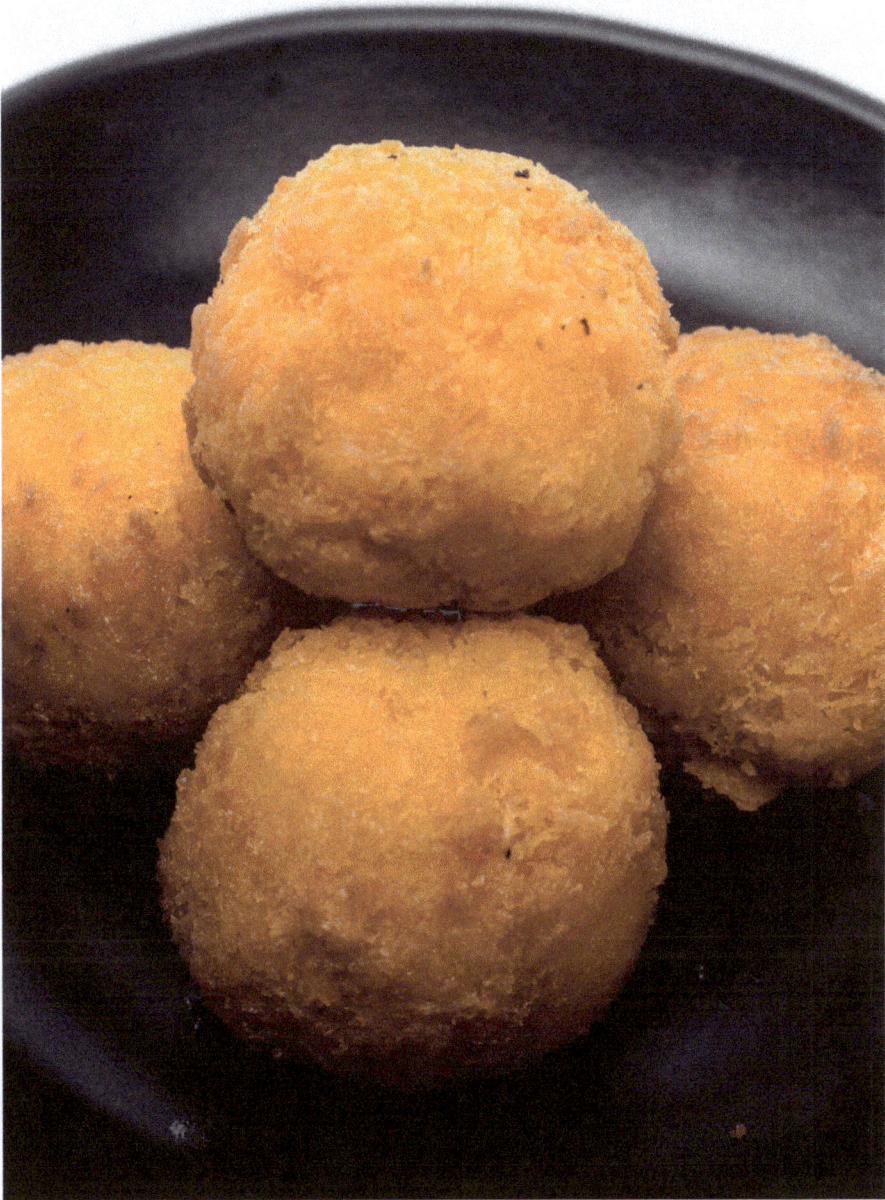

Ground Turkey Mini Meatloaves

Prep time: 10 minutes

Cook time: 30 minutes

Servings: 6

Ingredients

Lean ground turkey – 1 ½ pound

Onion – 1, diced

Celery – 2, diced

Bell pepper – 1, diced

Garlic – 4 cloves, minced

No-salt-added tomato sauce – 1 (8-ounce) can Egg white – 1

Salt-free bread crumbs – ¾ cup Molasses – 1 Tbsp.

Liquid smoke – ¼ tsp.

Freshly ground black pepper - ½ tsp. Salt-free ketchup – ¼ cup

Method

1. Preheat the oven to 375F. Spray a 6-cup muffin tin with oil and set aside.

2. Place all ingredients except for ketchup in a bowl and mix well.

3. Fill the muffin cups with the mixture and press in firmly.

4. Divide the ketchup between the muffin cups and spread evenly.

5. Place muffin tin on the middle rack in the oven and bake for 30 minutes.

6. Remove, cool, and serve.

Nutritional Facts Per Serving

Calories: 251

Fat: 7g

Carb: 21g

Protein: 25g

Sodium 112mg

Turkey and Brown Rice Stuffed Peppers

Prep time: 10 minutes

Cook time: 35 minutes

Servings: 4

Ingredients

Bell peppers – 4, core and seeded, leave the peppers intact

Lean ground turkey – 1 pound

Onion – 1, diced

Garlic – 3 cloves, minced

Celery – 2 stalks, diced

Cooked brown rice – 2 cups

No-salt-added diced tomatoes – 1 (15-ounce) can Salt-free tomato

paste – 2 Tbsp.

Seedless raisins – ¼ cup Ground cumin – 2 tsp.

Dried oregano – 1 tsp.

Ground cinnamon – ½ tsp.

Ground black pepper – ½ tsp.

Method

1.   Preheat the oven to 425F. Grease a baking pan with oil.

2.   Heat a pan over medium heat.

3.   Add onion, ground turkey, garlic, and celery and sauté for 5 minutes. Remove from heat.

4.   Add the remaining ingredients and mix.

5.   Fill each pepper with ¼ of the mixture. Pressing firmly to pack.

6.   Stand peppers in the prebaked baking pan, replace the pepper caps and then cover the pan with foil.

7.   Place in the middle rack in the oven and bake for 25 to 30 minutes, or until tender.

8.   Serve.

Nutritional Facts Per Serving

Calories: 354

Fat: 8g

Carb: 45g

Protein: 27g

Sodium 126mg

Grilled Tequila Chicken with Peppers

Prep time: 10 minutes

Cook time: 30 minutes

Servings: 4

Ingredientes

Lime juice – 1 cup

Tequila – 1/3 cup

Garlic – 3 cloves, chopped

Chopped fresh cilantro – ¼ cup

Agave nectar – 1 Tbsp.

Ground black pepper - ½ tsp.

Cumin – 1 tsp.

Ground coriander – ½ tsp.

Boneless, skinless chicken breasts – 4

Olive oil – 2 tsp.

Green bell pepper – 1, diced

Red bell pepper – 1, diced

Onion – 1, diced

Non-fat sour cream – ½ cup

Method

1.   In a bowl, add the lime juice, tequila garlic, cilantro, agave nectar, black pepper, cumin, and coriander and mix well.

2.   Add the chicken breasts and coat well. Cover and marinate in the for least 6 hours (in the refrigerator).

3.   Heat the grill. Cook the chicken for 10 to 15 minutes per side, or no longer pink.

4.   Meanwhile, heat the oil in a pan.

5.   Add the pepper and onion. Stir-fry for 5 minutes. Remove from heat. Remove chicken from grill.

6.   Serve with veggies and sour cream.

Nutritional Facts Per Serving

Calories: 259

Fat: 3g

Carb: 18g

Protein: 28g

Sodium 118mg

Orange-Rosemary Roasted Chicken

Prep time: 10 minutes

Cook time: 45 minutes

Servings: 6

Ingredients

Chicken breast halves – 3, skinless, bone-in, each 8 ounces
Chicken legs with thigh pieces – 3, skinless, bone-in, each 8 ounces

Garlic cloves – 2, minced Extra-virgin olive oil – 1 ½ tsp.

Fresh rosemary – 3 tsp.

Ground black pepper – 1/8 tsp.

Orange juice – ½ cup

Method

1.   Preheat oven at 450F. Grease a baking pan with cooking spray.

2.   Rub chicken with garlic, then with oil. Sprinkle with pepper and rosemary.

3.   Place the chicken pieces in the baking dish.

4.   Pour the orange juice.

5.   Cover and bake for 30 minutes, then flip the chicken with tongs and cook 10 to 15 minutes more or until browned. Baste the chicken with the pan juice from time to time.

6.   Serve chicken with pan juice.

Nutritional Facts Per Serving

Calories: 204

Fat: 8g

Carb: 2g

Protein: 31g

Sodium 95mg

Honey Crusted Chicken

Prep time: 10 minutes

Cook time: 25 minutes

Servings: 2

Ingredients

Saltine crackers – 8, (2-inch square each) crushed Paprika – 1 tsp.

Chicken breasts – 2, boneless, skinless (4-ounce each)

Honey – 4 tsp.

Cooking spray to grease a baking sheet

Method

1. Preheat the oven to 375F.

2. In a bowl, mix crushed crackers and paprika. Mix well.

3. In another bowl, add honey and chicken. Coat well.

4. Add to the cracker mixture and coat well.

5. Place the chicken in the prepared baking sheet.

6. Bake for 20 to 25 minutes.

7.   Serve.

Nutritional Facts Per Serving

Calories: 219

Fat: 3g

Carb: 21g

Protein: 27g

Sodium 187mg

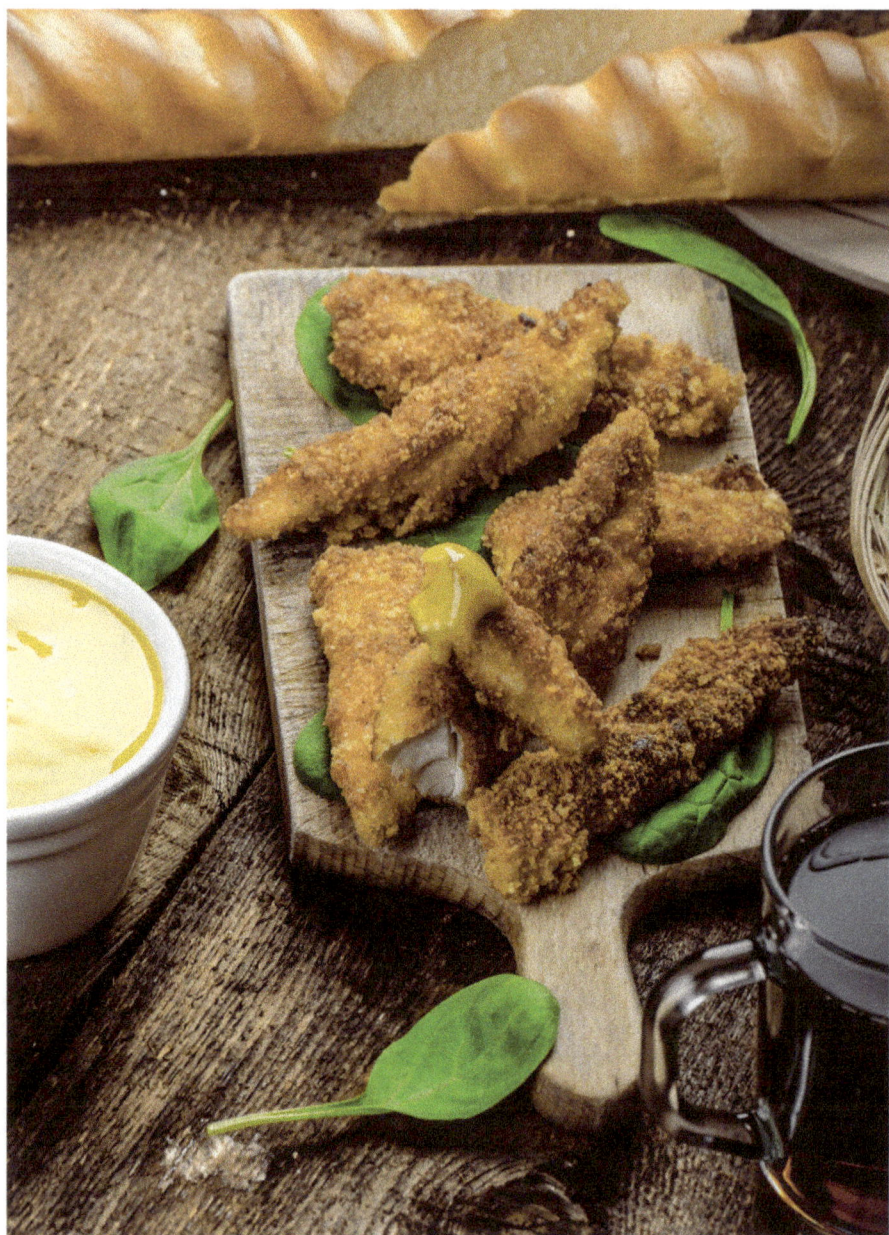

Italian Chicken and Vegetable

Prep time: 10 minutes

Cook time: 45 minutes

Servings: 1

Ingredients

Chicken breast – 1 skinless, boneless (3 ounces)

Diced zucchini – ½ cup

Diced potato – ½ cup

Diced onion – ¼ cup

Sliced baby carrots – ¼ cup

Sliced mushrooms – ¼ cup

Garlic powder – 1/8 tsp.

Italian seasoning – ¼ tsp.

Method

1.   Preheat oven to 350F.

2.   Grease a parchment paper with cooking spray.

3.   On the foil, add chicken, top mushrooms, carrots, onion, potato, and zucchini. Sprinkle with Italian seasoning and garlic powder.

4.   Fold the foil to make a packet.

5.   Place the packet on a cookie sheet.

6.   Bake until chicken and vegetables are tender, about 45 minutes.

7.   Serve.

Nutritional Facts Per Serving

Calories: 207

Fat: 2.5g

Carb: 23g

Protein: 23g

Sodium 72mg

Corn Spread

Serving: 4

Prep Time: 10 minutes

Cook Time: 10 minutes

Ingredients:

30-ounce canned corn, drained

2 green onions, chopped

½ cup coconut cream

1 jalapeno, chopped

½ teaspoon chili powder

How To:

1.   Take a pan and add corn, green onions, jalapeno, chili powder, stir well.

2.   Bring to a simmer over medium heat and cook for 10 minutes.

3.   Let it chill and add coconut cream.

4.   Stir well.

5. Serve and enjoy!

Nutrition (Per Serving)

Calories: 192

Fat: 5g

Carbohydrates: 11g

Protein: 8g

Moroccan Leeks Snack

Serving: 4

Prep Time: 10 minutes

Cook Time: nil

Ingredients:

1 bunch radish, sliced

3 cups leeks, chopped

1 ½ cups olives, pitted and sliced

Pinch turmeric powder

2 tablespoons essential olive oil

1 cup cilantro, chopped

How To:

1.   Take a bowl and mix in radishes, leeks, olives and cilantro.

2.   Mix well.

3.   Season with pepper, oil, turmeric and toss well.

4.   Serve and enjoy!

Nutrition (Per Serving)

Calories: 120

Fat: 1g

Carbohydrates: 1g

Protein: 6g

The Bell Pepper Fiesta

Serving: 4

Prep Time: 10 minutes

Cook Time: nil

Ingredients:

2 tablespoons dill, chopped

1 yellow onion, chopped

1 pound multi colored peppers, cut, halved, seeded and cut into thin strips

3 tablespoons organic olive oil

2 ½ tablespoons white wine vinegar Black pepper to taste

How To:

1.   Take a bowl and mix in sweet pepper, onion, dill, pepper, oil, vinegar and toss well.

2.   Divide between bowls and serve.

3.   Enjoy!

Nutrition (Per Serving)

Calories: 120

Fat: 3g

Carbohydrates: 1g

Protein: 6g

Spiced Up Pumpkin Seeds Bowls

Serving: 4

Prep Time: 10 minutes

Cook Time: 20 minutes

Ingredients:

½ tablespoon chili powder

½ teaspoon cayenne

2 cups pumpkin seeds

2 teaspoons lime juice

How To:

1.   Spread pumpkin seeds over lined baking sheet, add lime juice, cayenne and chili powder.

2.   Toss well.

3.   Pre-heat your oven to 275 degrees F.

4.   Roast in your oven for 20 minutes and transfer to small bowls.

5.   Serve and enjoy!

Nutrition (Per Serving)

Calories: 170

Fat: 3g

Carbohydrates: 10g

Protein: 6g

Mozzarella Cauliflower Bars

Serving: 4

Prep Time: 10 minutes

Cook Time: 40 minutes

Ingredients:

1 cauliflower head, riced

12 cup low-fat mozzarella cheese, shredded ¼ cup egg whites

1 teaspoon Italian dressing, low fat Pepper to taste

How To:

1.   Spread cauliflower rice over lined baking sheet.

2.   Pre-heat your oven to 375 degrees F.

3.   Roast for 20 minutes.

4.   Transfer to bowl and spread pepper, cheese, seasoning, egg whites and stir well.

5.   Spread in a rectangular pan and press.

6.   Transfer to oven and cook for 20 minutes more.

7.   Serve and enjoy!

Nutrition (Per Serving)

Calories: 140

Fat: 2g

Carbohydrates: 6g

Protein: 6g

Tomato Pesto Crackers

Serving: 4

Prep Time: 10 minutes

Cook Time: 15 minutes

Ingredients:

1 ¼ cups almond flour

½ teaspoon garlic powder

½ teaspoon baking powder

2 tablespoons sun-dried tomato Pesto

3 tablespoons ghee

½ teaspoon dried basil

¼ teaspoon pepper

How To:

1.   Pre-heat your oven to 325 degrees F.

2.   Take a bowl and add listed ingredients.

3.   Mix well and combine.

4.   Take a baking sheet lined with parchment paper and spread the dough.

5.   Transfer to oven and bake for 15 minutes. 6. Break into small sized crackers and serve.

6.   Enjoy!

Nutrition (Per Serving)

Calories: 204

Fat: 20g

Carbohydrates: 3g

Protein: 3g

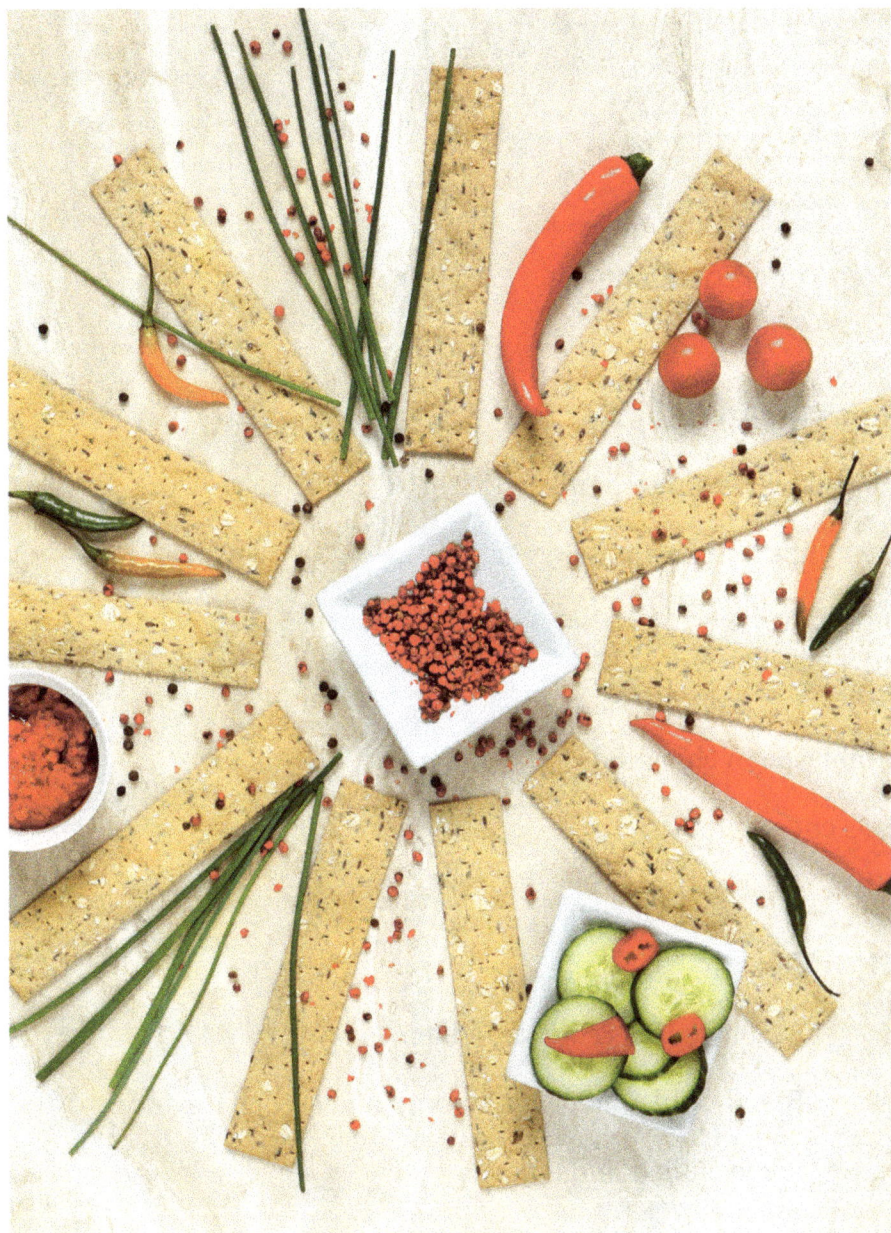

Green Delight

Serving: 1

Prep Time: 10 minutes

Ingredients:

¾ cup whole almond milk yogurt

2 ½ cups lettuce mix salad greens

1 pack stevia

1 tablespoon MCT oil

1 tablespoon chia seeds

1 ½ cups water

How To:

1.   Add listed ingredients to blender.

2.   Blend until you have a smooth and creamy texture.

3.   Serve chilled and enjoy!

Nutrition (Per Serving)

Calories: 320

Fat: 24g

Carbohydrates: 17g

Protein: 10g

Guilt Free Lemon and Rosemary Drink

Serving: 1

Prep Time: 10 minutes

Ingredients:

½ cup whole almond milk yogurt

1 cup garden greens

1 pack stevia

1 tablespoon olive oil

1 stalk fresh rosemary

1 tablespoon lemon juice, fresh

1 tablespoon pepitas

1 tablespoon flaxseed, ground

1 ½ cups water

How To:

1.   Add listed ingredients to blender.

2.   Blend until you have a smooth and creamy texture.

3.   Serve chilled and enjoy!

Nutrition (Per Serving)

Calories: 312

Fat: 25g

Carbohydrates: 14g

Protein: 9g

Strawberry and Rhubarb Smoothie

Serving: 1

Prep Time: 5 minutes

Cook Time: 3 minutes

Ingredients:

1 rhubarb stalk, chopped

1 cup fresh strawberries, sliced

½ cup plain Greek strawberries

Pinch of ground cinnamon

3 ice cubes

How To:

1.   Take a small saucepan and fill with water over high heat.

2.   Bring to boil and add rhubarb, boil for 3 minutes.

3.   Drain and transfer to a blender.

4.   Add strawberries, honey, yogurt, cinnamon and pulse

mixture until smooth.

5.   Add ice cubes and blend until thick with no lumps.

6.   Pour into glass and enjoy chilled.

Nutrition (Per Serving)

Calories: 295

Fat: 8g

Carbohydrates: 56g

Protein: 6g

Vanilla Hemp Drink

Serving: 1

Prep Time: 10 minutes

Ingredients:

1 cup water

1 cup unsweetened hemp almond milk, vanilla

1 ½ tablespoons coconut oil, unrefined

½ cup frozen blueberries, mixed

4 cups leafy greens, kale and spinach

1 tablespoon flaxseeds

1 tablespoon almond butter

How To:

1.   Add listed ingredients to blender.

2.   Blend until you have a smooth and creamy texture.

3.   Serve chilled and enjoy!

Nutrition (Per Serving)

Calories: 250

Fat: 20g

Carbohydrates: 10g

Protein: 7g

Yogurt and Kale Smoothie

Serving: 1

Prep Time: 10 minutes

Ingredients:

1 cup whole almond milk yogurt

1 cup baby kale greens

1 pack stevia

1 tablespoon MCT oil

1 tablespoons sunflower seeds

1 cup water

How To:

1.   Add listed ingredients to blender 2. Blend until you have a smooth and creamy texture

2.   Serve chilled and enjoy!

Nutrition (Per Serving)

Calories: 329

Fat: 26g

Carbohydrates: 15g

Protein: 11g

Baby Potatoes

Serving: 4

Prep Time: 10 minutes

Cook Time: 35 minutes

Ingredients:

2 pounds new yellow potatoes, scrubbed and cut into wedges

2 tablespoons extra virgin olive oil

2 teaspoons fresh rosemary, chopped

1 teaspoon garlic powder

½ teaspoon freshly ground black pepper and sunflower seeds

How To:

1.   Pre-heat your oven to 400 degrees F.

2.   Line a baking sheet with aluminum foil and set it aside.

3.   Take a large bowl and add potatoes, olive oil, garlic, rosemary, sea sunflower seeds and pepper.

4.   Spread potatoes in a single layer on a baking sheet and bake for 35 minutes.

5.   Serve and enjoy!

Nutrition (Per Serving)

Calories: 225

Fat: 7g

Carbohydrates: 37g

Protein: 5g

Cauliflower Cakes

Serving: 4

Prep Time: 10 minutes

Cook Time: 10 minutes

Ingredients:

4 cups cauliflowers, cut into florets

1 cup kite ricotta/cashew cheese, grated

2 eggs, lightly beaten

1 teaspoon paprika

1 teaspoon chili powder

Sunflower seeds and pepper to taste

½ cup fresh parsley, chopped

1 tablespoon olive oil

How To:

1.   Add cauliflower, cheese, paprika, eggs, chili, sunflower seeds, pepper and parsley into a large sized bowl.

2.   Mix well.

3.	Drizzle olive oil into frying pan and place over medium-high heat.

4.	Shape cauliflower mixture into 12 even patties.

5.	Once oil is hot, fry cakes until both sides are golden brown.

6.	Serve hot and enjoy!

Nutrition (Per Serving)

Calories: 180

Fat: 8g

Carbohydrates: 6g

Protein: 8g

Tender Coconut and Cauliflower Rice with Chili

Serving: 4

Prep Time: 20 minutes

Cook Time: 20 minutes

Ingredients:

3 cups cauliflower, riced

2/3 cups full-fat coconut almond milk

1-2 teaspoons sriracha paste

¼- ½ teaspoon onion powder

Sunflower seeds as needed

Fresh basil for garnish

How To:

1.   Take a pan and place it over medium low heat.

2.   Add all of the ingredients and stir them until fully combined.

3.   Cook for about 5-10 minutes, making sure that the lid is on.

4.   Remove the lid and keep cooking until any excess liquid is absorbed.

5.   Once the rice is soft and creamy, enjoy!

Nutrition (Per Serving)

Calories: 95

Fat: 7g

Carbohydrates: 4g

Protein: 1g

Apple Slices

Serving: 4

Prep Time: 10 minutes

Cook Time: 10 minutes

Ingredients:

1 cup of coconut oil

¼ cup date paste

2 tablespoons ground cinnamon

4 Granny Smith apples, peeled and sliced, cored

How To:

1. Take a large sized skillet and place it over medium heat.

2. Add oil and allow the oil to heat up.

3. Stir cinnamon and date paste into the oil.

4. Add sliced apples and cook for 5-8 minutes until crispy.

5. Serve and enjoy!

Nutrition (Per Serving)

Calories: 368

Fat: 23g

Carbohydrates: 44g

Protein: 1g

The Exquisite Spaghetti Squash

Serving: 6

Prep Time: 5 minutes

Cooking Time: 7-8 hours

Ingredients:

1 spaghetti squash

2 cups water

How To:

1.   Wash squash carefully with water and rinse it well.

2.   Puncture 5-6 holes in the squash using a fork.

3.   Place squash in Slow Cooker.

4.   Place lid and cook on LOW for 7-8 hours.

5.   Remove squash to cutting board and let it cool.

6.   Cut squash in half and discard seeds.

7.   Use two forks and scrape out squash strands and transfer to bowl.

8.   Serve and enjoy!

Nutrition (Per Serving)

Calories: 52

Fat: 0g

Carbohydrates: 12g

Protein: 1g

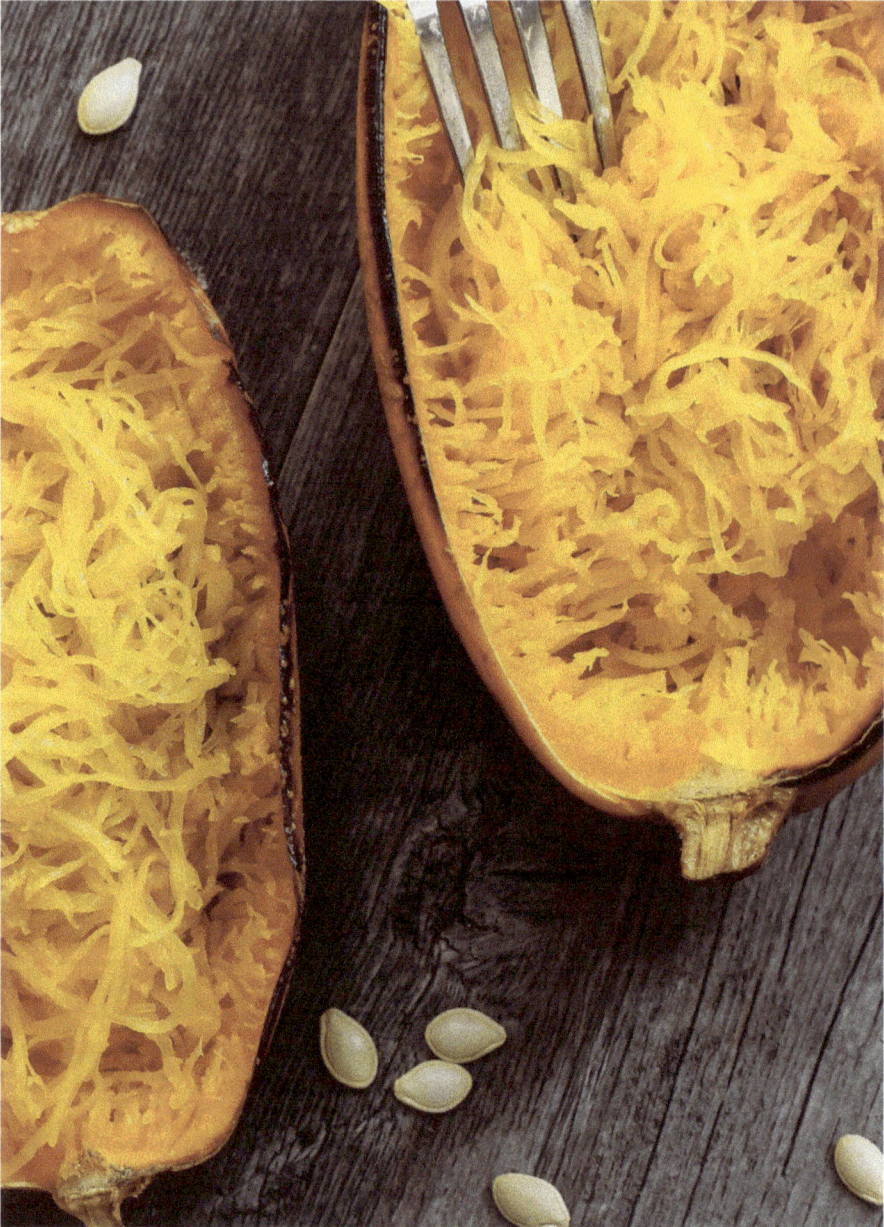

Vanilla Sweet Potato Porridge

Serving: 5

Prep Time: 10 minutes

Cook Time: 8 hours

Ingredients:

6 sweet potatoes, peeled and cut into 1-inch cubes

1 ½ cups light coconut milk

1 teaspoon ground cinnamon

1 teaspoon ground cardamom

1 teaspoon pure vanilla extract

1 cup raisins Pinch of salt

How To:

1.   Add sweet potatoes coconut milk, vanilla, cardamom, cinnamon to your Slow Cooker.

2.   Close lid and cook on LOW for 8 hours.

3.   Open the lid and mash the entire mixture using potato masher to mash the sweet potatoes, stir well.

4.   Stir in raisins, salt and serve.

5.   Serve and enjoy!

Nutrition (Per Serving)

Calories: 317

Fat: 4g

Carbohydrates: 71g

Protein: 4g

A Nice German Oatmeal

Serving: 3

Prep Time: 10 minutes

Cook Time: 8 hours

Ingredients:

1 cup steel-cut oats

3 cups water

6 ounces coconut milk

2 tablespoons cocoa powder

1 tablespoon brown sugar

1 tablespoon coconut, shredded

How to

1. Grease the Slow Cooker well.

2. Add the listed ingredients to your Cooker and stir.

3. Place lid and cook on LOW for 8 hours.

4. Divide amongst serving bowls and enjoy!

Nutrition (Per Serving)

Calories: 200

Fat: 4g

Carbohydrates: 11g

Protein: 5g

Very Nutty Banana Oatmeal

Serving: 4

Prep Time: 15 minutes

Cook Time: 7-9 hours

Ingredients:

1 cup steel-cut oats

1 ripe banana, mashed

2 cups unsweetened almond milk

1 cup water

1 ½ tablespoons honey

½ teaspoon vanilla extract

¼ cup almonds, chopped

1 teaspoon ground cinnamon

¼ teaspoon ground nutmeg

How To:

1.   Grease the Slow Cooker well.

2. Add the listed ingredients to your Slow Cooker and stir.

3. Cover with lid and cook on LOW for 7-9 hours.

4. Serve and enjoy!

Nutrition (Per Serving)

Calories: 230

Fat: 7g

Carbohydrates: 40g

Protein: 5g

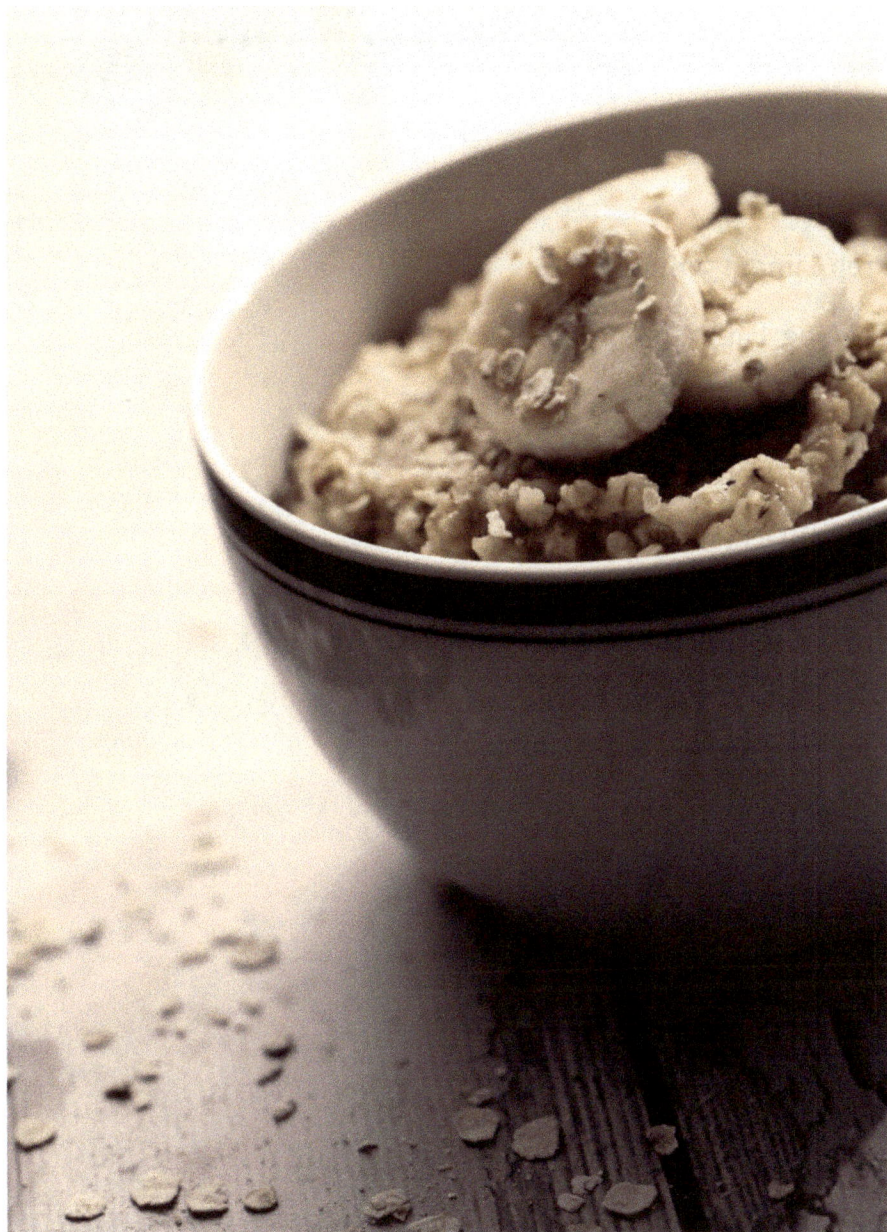

Cool Coconut Flatbread

Serving: 4

Prep Time: 15 minutes

Cooking Time: 10 minutes

Ingredients:

1 ½ tablespoons coconut flour

¼ teaspoon baking powder

1/8 teaspoon sunflower seeds

1 tablespoon coconut oil, melted

1 whole egg

How To:

1.   Preheat your oven to 350 degrees F.

2.   Add coconut flour, leaven , sunflower seeds.

3.   Add copra oil , eggs and stir well until mixed.

4.   Leave the batter for several minutes.

5.   Pour half the batter onto the baking pan.

6. Spread it to make a circle, repeat with remaining batter.

7. Bake within the oven for 10 minutes.

8. Once you get a golden-brown texture, let it cool and serve.

9. Enjoy!

Nutrition (Per Serving)

Total Carbs: 9 (%)

Fiber: 3g

Protein: 8g (%)

Fat: 20g (%)

Perfect Homemade Pickled Ginger

Gari

Serving: 8

Prep Time: 40 minutes

Cook Time: 5 minutes

Ingredients:

About 8 ounces of fresh ginger root, completely peeled

1 teaspoon and extra ½ teaspoon of fine sunflower seeds

1 cup vinegar, rice

1/3 cup sugar, white

How To:

1.   Cut your ginger into small-sized chunks and transfer them to a bowl.

2.   Season with sunflower seeds and stir, let the mixture sit for a minimum of half-hour .

3.   Take a saucepan and add sugar and vinegar, heat it up, bring the mixture to a boil and keep boiling until the sugar has

completely dissolved.

4.   Pour the liquid over your ginger pieces.

5.   Let it cool and wait until the water changes color.

6.   Enjoy!

7.   Alternatively, store in jars and use as required.

Nutrition (Per Serving)

Calories: 14

Fat: 0.1g

Carbohydrates: 3g

Protein: 0.1g

Avocado and Blueberry Medley

Serving: 4

Prep Time: 5 minutes

Cook Time: Nil

Ingredients:

1 frozen banana

2 avocados, quartered

2 cups berries

Maple syrup as needed

How To:

1.   Take your blender and add all ingredients except syrup.

2.   Add drinking water and blend.

3.   Garnish with syrup and pour in smoothie glasses.

4.   Enjoy!

Nutrition (Per Serving)

Calories: 250

Fat: 13g

Carbohydrates: 40g

Protein 4g

Healthy Zucchini Stir Fry

Serving: 4

Prep Time: 10 minutes

Cook Time: 10 minutes

Ingredients:

2 heaped tablespoons olive oil

1 medium-sized onion, sliced thinly

2 medium-sized zucchini, cut up into thin sized strips

2 heaped tablespoons teriyaki flavored sauce, low sodium

1 tablespoon coconut aminos

1 tablespoon sesame seed, toasted Ground pepper (black) as much as needed

How To:

1.   Take a skillet and place it over medium level heat.

2.   Add onions, and stir-cook for five minutes.

3.   Add your zucchini and stir-cook for 1 minute more.

4.   Gently add the sauces alongside the sesame seeds.

5.   Cook for five minutes more until the zucchini are soft.

6.   Finally, add the pepper and enjoy!

Nutrition (Per Serving)

Calories: 110

Fat: 9g

Carbohydrates: 8g

Protein: 3g

Greek Lemon Chicken Bowl

Serving: 6

Prep Time: 10 minutes

Cook Time: 15 minutes

Ingredients:

2 cups chicken, cooked and chopped

2 cans chicken broth, fat free

2 medium carrots, chopped

¼ teaspoon pepper

2 tablespoons parsley, snipped

¼ cup lemon juice

1 can cream chicken soup, fat free, low sodium ½ cup onion, chopped

1 garlic clove, minced

How To:

1.   Take a pot and add all the ingredients except parsley into it.
2.

2.   Season with salt and pepper.

3.   Bring the combination to a overboil medium-high heat.

4.   Reduce the warmth and simmer for quarter-hour .

5.   Garnish with parsley.

6.   Serve hot and enjoy!

Nutrition (Per Serving)

Calories: 520

Fat: 33g

Carbohydrates: 31g

Protein: 30g

Chilled Chicken, Artichoke and Zucchini Platter

Serving: 4

Prep Time: 10 minutes

Cook Time: 5 minutes

Ingredients:

2 medium chicken breasts, cooked and cut into 1-inch cubes ¼ cup extra virgin olive oil

2 cups artichoke hearts, drained and roughly chopped

3 large zucchini, diced/cut into small rounds

1 can (15 ounce) chickpeas

1 cup Kalamata olives

½ teaspoon Fresh ground black pepper

½ teaspoon Italian seasoning

¼ cup parmesan, grated

How To:

1.   Take an outsized skillet and place it over medium heat, heat up vegetable oil.

2.   Add zucchini and sauté for five minutes, season with salt and pepper.

3.   Remove from heat and add all the listed ingredients to the skillet.

4.   Stir until combined.

5.   Transfer to glass container and store.

6.   Serve and enjoy!

Nutrition (Per Serving)

Calories: 457

Fat: 22g

Carbohydrates: 30g

Protein: 24g

Chicken and Carrot Stew

Serving: 6

Prep Time: 15 minutes

Cook Time: 6 hours

Ingredients:

4 chicken breasts, boneless and cubed

2 cups chicken broth

1 cup tomatoes, chopped

3 cups carrots, peeled and cubed

1 teaspoon thyme dried

1 cup onion, chopped

2 garlic cloves, minced

Pepper to taste

How To:

1.   Add all the ingredients to the Slow Cooker.

2.   Stir and shut the lid.

3.   Cook for six hours.

4.   Serve hot and enjoy!

Nutrition (Per Serving)

Calories: 182

Fat: 4g

Carbohydrates: 10g

Protein: 39g

Tasty Spinach Pie

Serving: 2

Prep Time: 10 minutes

Cooking Time: 4 hours

Ingredients:

10 ounces spinach

2 cups baby Bella mushrooms, chopped

1 red bell pepper, chopped

1 ½ cups low-fat cheese, shredded

8 whole eggs

1 cup coconut cream

2 tablespoons chives, chopped

Pinch of pepper

½ cup almond flour

¼ teaspoon baking soda

How To:

1.   Take a bowl and add eggs, coconut milk , chives, pepper and whisk well.

2.   Add almond flour, bicarbonate of soda , cheese, mushrooms bell pepper, spinach and toss well.

3.   Grease your cooker and transfer mix to the Slow Cooker.

4.   Place lid and cook on LOW for 4 hours.

5.   Slice and enjoy!

Nutrition (Per Serving)

Calories: 201

Fat: 6g

Carbohydrates: 8g

Protein: 5g

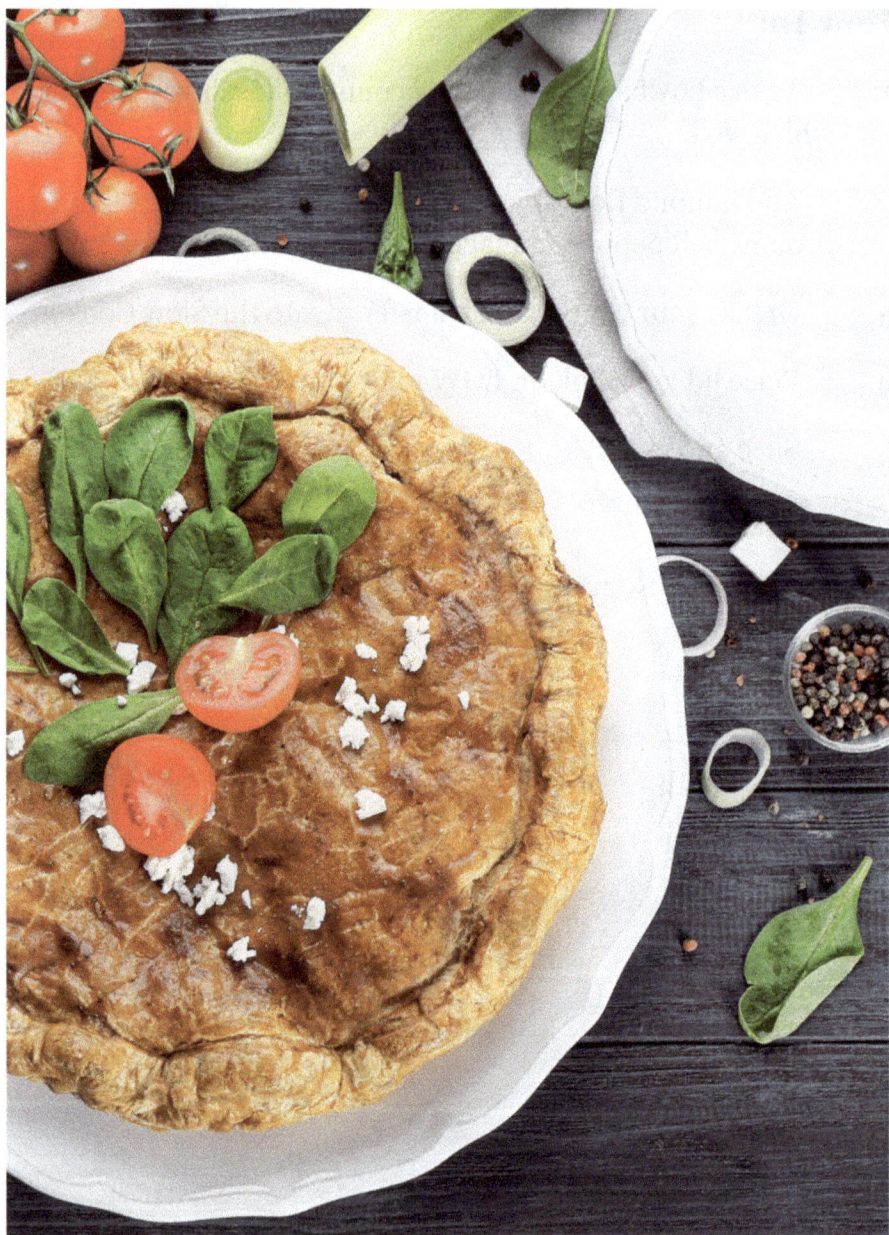

Mesmerizing Carrot and Pineapple Mix

Serving: 10

Prep Time: 10 minutes

Cooking Time: 6 hours

Ingredients:

1 cup raisins 6 cups water

23 ounces natural applesauce

2 tablespoons stevia

2 tablespoons cinnamon powder

14 ounces carrots, shredded

8 ounces canned pineapple, crushed

1 tablespoon pumpkin pie spice

How To:

1. Add carrots, applesauce, raisins, stevia, cinnamon, pineapple, pie spice to your Slow Cooker and gently stir.

2.   Place lid and cook on LOW for six hours.

3.   Serve and enjoy!

Nutrition (Per Serving)

Calories: 179

Fat: 5g

Carbohydrates: 15g

Protein: 4g

Ethiopian Cabbage Delight

Serving: 6

Prep Time: 15 minutes

Cook Time: 6- 8 hours

Ingredients:

½ cup water

1 head green cabbage, cored and chopped

1-pound sweet potatoes, peeled and chopped

3 carrots, peeled and chopped

1 onion, sliced

1 teaspoon extra virgin olive oil

½ teaspoon ground turmeric

½ teaspoon ground cumin

¼ teaspoon ground ginger

How To:

1.   Add water to your Slow Cooker.

2.   Take a medium bowl and add cabbage, carrots, sweet potatoes, onion and blend.

3.   Add vegetable oil, turmeric, ginger, cumin and toss until the veggies are fully coated.

4.   Transfer veggie mix to your Slow Cooker.

5.   Cover and cook on LOW for 6-8 hours.

6.   Serve and enjoy!

Nutrition (Per Serving)

Calories: 155

Fat: 2g

Carbohydrates: 35g

Protein: 4g

The Vegan Lovers Refried Beans

Serving: 12

Prep Time: 5 minutes

Cook Time: 10 hours

Ingredients:

4 cups vegetable broth

4 cups water

3 cups dried pinto beans

1 onion, chopped

2 jalapeno peppers, minced

4 garlic cloves, minced

1 tablespoon chili powder

2 teaspoon ground cumin

1 teaspoon sweet paprika

1 teaspoon salt

½ teaspoon fresh ground black pepper

How To:

1.   Add the listed ingredients to your Slow Cooker.

2.   Cover and cook on HIGH for 10 hours.

3.   If there's any extra liquid, ladle the liquid up and reserve it during a bowl.

4.   Use an immersion blender to blend the mixture (in the Slow Cooker) until smooth.

5.   Add the reserved liquid.

6.   Serve hot and enjoy!

Nutrition (Per Serving)

Calories: 91

Fat: 0g

Carbohydrates: 16g

Protein: 5g

Cool Apple and Carrot Harmony

Serving: 6

Prep Time: 10 minutes

Cook Time: 10 minutes

Ingredients:

1 cup apple juice

1 pound baby carrots

1 tablespoon cornstarch

1 tablespoon mint, chopped

How To:

1.   Add fruit juice, carrots, cornstarch and mint to your Instant Pot.

2.   Stir and lock the lid.

3.   Cook on high for 10 minutes.

4.   Perform a fast release.

5.   Divide the combination amongst plates and serve.

6.   Enjoy!

Nutrition (Per Serving)

Calories: 161

Fat: 2g

Carbohydrates: 9g

Protein: 8g

Mac and Chokes

Serving: 6

Prep Time: 5 minutes

Cook Time: 20 minutes

Ingredients:

1 tablespoon of olive oil

1 large sized diced onion

10 minced garlic cloves

1 can artichoke hearts

1-pound uncooked macaroni shells

12-ounce baby spinach

4 cups vegetable broth

1 teaspoon red pepper flakes

4 ounces vegan cheese

¼ cup cashew cream

How To:

1.   Set the pot to Sauté mode and add oil, allow the oil to heat up and add onions.

2.   Cook for two minutes.

3.   Add garlic and stir well.

4.   Add artichoke hearts and sauté for 1 minute more.

5.   Add uncooked pasta and three cups of broth alongside 2 cups of water.

6.   Mix well.

7.   Lock the lid and cook on high for 4 minutes.

8.   Quick release the pressure.

9.   Open the pot and stir.

10.   Add extra water, fold in spinach and cook on Sauté mode for a couple of minutes.

11.   Add cashew cream and grated vegan cheese.

12.   Add pepper flakes and blend well.

13.   Enjoy!

Nutrition (Per Serving)

Calories: 649

Fat: 29g

Carbohydrates: 64g

Protein: 34g

Bay Scallop Chowder

Serving: 4

Prep Time: 10 minutes

Cook Time: 18 minutes

Ingredients:

1 medium onion, chopped

2 ½ cups chicken stock

4 slices bacon, chopped

3 cups daikon radish, chopped

½ teaspoon dried thyme

2 cups low-fat cream

1 tablespoon almond butter

Pepper to taste

1 pound bay scallops

How To:

1.   Heat olive over medium heat in a large sized saucepan, add bacon and cook until crisp, add onion and daikon radish.

2.   Cook for 5 minutes, add chicken stock.

3.   Simmer for 8 minutes, season with salt and pepper, thyme.

4. Add heavy cream, bay scallops, simmer for 4 minutes

5.   Serve and enjoy!

Nutrition (Per Serving)

Calories: 307

Fat: 22g

Carbohydrates: 7g

Protein: 22g

Salmon and Vegetable Soup

Serving: 4

Prep Time: 10 minutes

Cook Time: 22 minutes

Ingredients:

2 tablespoons extra-virgin olive oil

1 leek, chopped

1 red onion, chopped

Pepper to taste

2 carrots, chopped

4 cups low stock vegetable stock

4 ounces salmon, skinless and boneless, cubed ½ cup coconut cream

1 tablespoon dill, chopped

How To:

1.   Take a pan and place it over medium heat, add leek, onion, stir and cook for 7 minutes.

2. Add pepper, carrots, stock and stir.

3. Boil for 10 minutes.

4. Add salmon, cream, dill and stir.

5. Boil for 5-6 minutes.

6. Ladle into bowls and serve.

7. Enjoy!

Nutrition (Per Serving)

Calories: 240

Fat: 4g

Carbohydrates: 7g

Protein: 12g

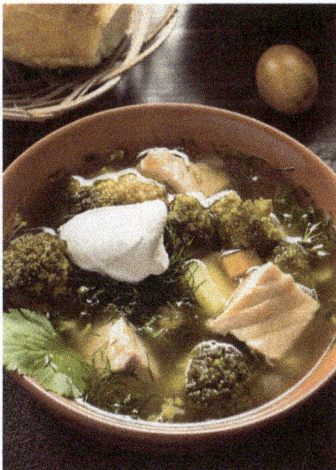

Garlic Tomato Soup

Serving: 4

Prep Time: 15 minutes

Cook Time: 15 minutes

Ingredients:

Roma tomatoes, chopped

1 cup tomatoes, sundried

2 tablespoons coconut oil

5 garlic cloves, chopped

14 ounces coconut milk

1 cup vegetable broth

Pepper to taste

Basil, for garnish

How To:

1.   Take a pot, heat oil into it.

2.   Sauté the garlic in it for ½ minute.

3.   Mix in the Roma tomatoes and cook for 8-10 minutes.

4.   Stir occasionally.

5.   Add in the rest of the ingredients, except the basil, and stir well.

6.   Cover the lid and cook for 5 minutes.

7.   Let it cool.

8.   Blend the soup until smooth by using an immersion blender.

9.   Garnish with basil.

10.   Serve and enjoy!

Nutrition (Per Serving)

Calories: 240

Fat: 23g

Carbohydrates: 16g

Protein: 7g

Melon Soup

Serving: 4

Prep Time:6 minutes

Cook Time: Nil

Ingredients:

4 cups casaba melon, seeded and cubed

1 tablespoon fresh ginger, grated

¾ cup coconut milk Juice of 2 limes

How To:

Add the lime juice, coconut milk, casaba melon, ginger and salt into your blender.

Blend for 1-2 minutes until you get a smooth mixture.

Serve and enjoy!

Nutrition (Per Serving)

Calories: 134

Fat: 9g

Carbohydrates: 13g

Protein: 2g

Spring Salad

Serving: 2

Prep Time: 10-15 minutes

Cook Time: 0 minutes

Ingredients:

2 ounces mixed green vegetables

3 tablespoons roasted pine nuts

2 tablespoons 5-minute 5 Keto Raspberry Vinaigrette

2 tablespoons shaved Parmesan

2 slices bacon

Pepper as required

How To:

1.   Take a cooking pan and add bacon, cook the bacon until crispy.

2.   Take a bowl and add the salad ingredients and mix well, add crumbled bacon into the salad.

3.   Mix well.

4.   Dress it with your favorite dressing.

5.   Enjoy!

Nutrition (Per Serving)

Calories: 209

Fat: 17g

Net Carbohydrates: 10g

Protein: 4g

Hearty Orange and Onion Salad

Serving: 2

Prep Time: 10 minutes

Cook Time: nil

Ingredients:

6 large oranges

3 tablespoons red wine vinegar

6 tablespoons olive oil

1 teaspoon dried oregano

1 red onion, thinly sliced

1 cup olive oil

¼ cup fresh chives, chopped Ground black pepper

How To:

1.   Peel orange and cut into 4-5 crosswise slices.

2.   Transfer orange to shallow dish.

3.   Drizzle vinegar, olive oil on top.

4.   Sprinkle oregano.

5.   Toss well to mix.

6.   Chill for 30 minutes and arrange sliced onion and black olives on top.

7.   Sprinkle more chives and pepper.

8.   Serve and enjoy!

Nutrition (Per Serving)

Calories: 120

Fat: 6g

Carbohydrates: 20g

Protein: 2g

Ground Beef Bell Peppers

Serving: 3

Prep Time: 10 minutes

Cook Time: 10 minutes

Ingredients:

1 onion, chopped

2 tablespoons coconut oil

1 pound ground beef

1 red bell pepper, diced

2 cups spinach, chopped

Pepper to taste

How To:

1.   Take a skillet and place it over medium heat.

2.   Add onion and cook until slightly browned.

3.   Add spinach and ground beef.

4.   Stir fry until done.

5.   Take the mixture and fill up the bell peppers.

6.   Serve and enjoy!

Nutrition (Per Serving)

Calories: 350

Fat: 23g

Carbohydrates: 4g

Protein: 28g

Foiled Fish

Serving: 4

Prep Time: 20 minutes

Cook Time: 40 minutes

Ingredients:

2 rainbow trout fillets

tablespoon olive oil

teaspoon garlic salt

1 teaspoon ground black pepper

1 fresh jalapeno pepper, sliced

1 lemon, sliced

How To:

1.   Pre-heat your oven to 400 degrees F.

2.   Rinse your fish and pat them dry.

3.   Rub the fillets with olive oil, season with some garlic salt and black pepper.

4. Place each of your seasoned fillets on a large sized sheet of aluminum foil.

5. Top it with some jalapeno slices and squeeze the juice from your lemons over your fish.

6. Arrange the lemon slices on top of your fillets.

7. Carefully seal up the edges of your foil and form a nice enclosed packet.

8. Place your packets on your baking sheet.

9. Bake them for about 20 minutes.

10. Once the flakes start to flake off with a fork, the fish is ready!

Nutrition (Per Serving)

Calories: 213

Fat: 10g

Carbohydrates: 8g

Protein: 24g

Brazilian Shrimp Stew

Serving: 4

Prep Time: 20 minutes

Cook Time: 25 minutes

Ingredients:

Tablespoons lime juice

1 ½ tablespoons cumin, ground

½ tablespoons paprika

½ teaspoons garlic, minced

½ teaspoons pepper

Pounds tilapia fillets, cut into bits

1 large onion, chopped

Large bell peppers, cut into strips

1 can (14 ounces) tomato, drained

1 can (14 ounces) coconut milk handful of cilantros, chopped

How To:

1.   Take a large sized bowl and add lime juice, cumin, paprika, garlic, pepper and mix well.

2.   Add tilapia and coat it up.

3.   Cover and allow to marinate for 20 minutes.

4.   Set your Instant Pot to Sauté mode and add olive oil.

5.   Add onions and cook for 3 minutes until tender.

6.   Add pepper strips, tilapia, and tomatoes to a skillet.

7.   Pour coconut milk and cover, simmer for 20 minutes.

8.   Add cilantro during the final few minutes.

9.   Serve and enjoy!

Nutrition (Per Serving)

Calories: 471

Fat: 44g

Carbohydrates: 13g

Protein: 12g

www.ingramcontent.com/pod-product-compliance
Lightning Source LLC
Chambersburg PA
CBHW050748030426
42336CB00012B/1710